Contents

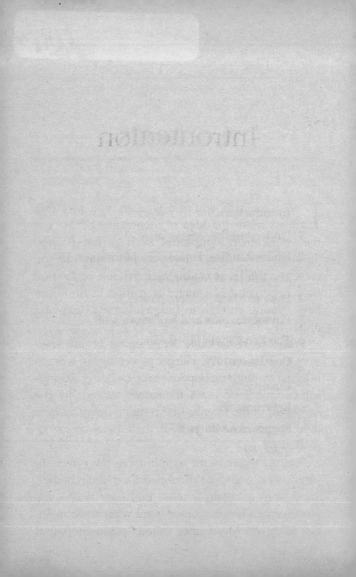

Introduction

Let's face it. If you're a woman, you probably don't relish the idea of menopause. There are the well-known symptoms, such as hot flashes, night sweats, vaginal dryness, and bone-thinning osteoporosis. There is also the inevitable realization that menopause is a major transition in life, from being young enough to bear children to growing older.

With the remarkable lengthening of life span over the past century, a larger percentage of women is living through menopause and spending a significant number of years thereafter. Indeed, by the early part of the twenty-first century, many women may spend close to half of their lives as menopausal.

Women today want to minimize the effects of menopause and post-menopause on their bodies. They want to retain a sense that their bodies are younger. In a sense, women want what anthropologist Margaret Mead once called "postmenopausal zest," and they want it safely—without dangerous drugs.

Pharmaceutical companies, however, are eager to sell women estrogen, either in the form of a synthetic compound or that derived from the urine of pregnant horses. Women who take such drugs should know about the side effects, such as excessive bleeding and pain, and the long-term risks, including a greater chance of developing breast cancer. There *are* natural and safe alternatives, which are the subject of this book.

Most plants produce their own versions of estrogens, called "phytoestrogens," which means "plant estrogens." These naturally occurring estrogen-like compounds help the body manage its own hormones by keeping the levels of these hormones more stable.

For example, Japanese women who eat a traditional diet consume large quantities of phytoestrogens; not surprisingly, there is no term in the Japanese language that corresponds to "hot flashes." It seems that Japanese women typically don't experience menopausal hot flashes to any great extent. In contrast, the typical American woman obtains just a fraction of the phytoestrogens that women in Japan eat. In large part, this is due to the fact that the typical American diet contains few of the plant foods that are rich in phytoestrogens. The other reason is that food processing removes many of the phytoestrogens that are normally found in food. The Western diet relies heavily on processed foods. You can counter this disadvantage by eating a more natural diet, opting for the convenience of dietary supplements containing various phytoestrogens, or doing both.

This book, *All About Menopause, Phytoestrogens, and Red Clover* explains exactly what menopause is and what life can be like during menopause and post-menopause. The questions are likely those that you've wanted to ask your doctor but never have had the opportunity. This book also tells you all about remarkable, natural, and safe phytoestrogens. It focuses on red clover, a humble plant that is one of the richest source of phytoestrogens in nature, and explains how you can use it to feel like the woman you want to.

1.

Understanding Menopause

Once, not too many years ago, women were embarrassed to mention the word menopause in public. Those days are gone, as is the idea that menopause is the beginning of the end for women. Menopause is not a disease; it's a natural process in what is becoming an unnatural world. If you're like most middle-aged women, you want to know more about menopause— more than your doctor has time to explain. In this first chapter, we cover some of the basics about menopause.

Q. What is menopause?

A. Menopause is a perfectly natural event for women. It certainly is not a disease. It simply represents a stage of life when women make a transition from being fertile to infertile; ovulation ceases at this point. With no further eggs being produced and released, menstruation also ceases.

There has been a suggestion in recent years that menopause is a modern phenomenon and that women were never designed to live long enough to experience menopause. On the contrary, menopause has always been a fact of life. In fact, it has been written about for thousands of years. As far back as 350 B.C., Aristotle noted that menstruation stops at about age forty. Because life expectancy was considerably shorter until relatively recently, it was not every woman who lived to see menopause. However, menopause is not for that reason an aberration.

The older term for this change of life is "climacteric," which comes from ancient Greek and signifies the steps of a ladder. The more modern term comes from French and literally means a *pause* from *menstruation*.

Q. What causes menopause?

A. Menopause occurs because ovulation stops, and ovulation stops when estrogen levels fall below a certain level.

Estrogen is produced in a woman's ovaries and its main function in the body is to maintain the female reproductive system in full functioning order. A woman is normally aware of the effect of estrogen on her body because of her monthly period, or menstruation. Throughout a woman's childbearing years, her two ovaries are constantly making a relatively steady amount of estrogen, although the amount does fluctuate through the course of the monthly menstrual cycle.

From approximately age thirty-five onward, the body starts to decrease its estrogen production. Women start to become aware of this change in their bodies through changes in their monthly cycles. Because one of the major effects of estrogen is to thicken the lining of the uterus, this thickening decreases as estrogen levels decline. This translates into changes in the monthly period. They can become less regular, shorter, or less heavy in terms of blood flow. The estrogen level finally falls to a point where menstruation doesn't occur anymore and the body enters menopause.

Q. Why do a woman's estrogen levels decline?

A. Each of your two ovaries contains a great number of immature eggs known as follicles. Each follicle has the potential to develop into a mature egg, but the vast majority never make it to this stage. Out of the million or so potential eggs a girl is born with, no more than several hundred will ever fully develop. Each month only one, or occasionally two, of the follicles will develop into a mature egg. Whether or not these follicles ever develop into mature eggs, they all make a small amount of estrogen. And the minute contribution from each of these thousands of follicles adds up to a considerable amount of estrogen.

From an early age, however, there is a progressive loss of follicles. The follicles literally die off at the rate of thousands per month. So, from a total number of about 1 million at birth, one is left with several hundred thousand egg follicles by puberty. By the time a woman reaches her mid-forties, there are only about a thousand or so left. By the time a woman reaches her late forties or early fifties, the estrogen output from the remaining follicles is just too low to support menstruation.

Q. At what age does menopause begin?

A. This varies considerably between women. The stage at which estrogen levels drop enough to start seeing a change in the monthly period is known as the perimenopause. This literally means the time around the menopause. The perimenopause can start as early as the mid-thirties or as late as the mid-fifties, but usually it starts in the early-to-mid-forties. The years between the time a woman first notices some irregularity in her periods and the time they completely stop define perimenopause. This period can last from one to ten years but usually lasts about five years. Menopause itself, consequently, can happen any time under natural conditions from the early forties to the late fifties, but, in most cases, it happens between forty-eight and fifty-three years of age.

As signs of the beginning of perimenopause, a woman may notice that her periods are becoming lighter, changing their lengths (either shortening or lengthening), or becoming less regular to the point where some months may go by without a period happening at all. The times between the periods eventually start to stretch into several months and finally the periods stop altogether. This natural process can be caused at a younger age by what doctors call "surgical menopause," which is usually the result of a hysterectomy.

2.

Understanding Female Sex Hormones

Women make a number of different sex hormones. They usually are classified either as female sex hormones (estrogens and progesterone) or male sex hormone (testosterone). The terms "female" and "male" are a bit misleading because men also make female sex hormones, just as women also make male sex hormones. Both types of sex hormones play important roles in both sexes. In this chapter, however, we'll concentrate on the basic functions of the female sex hormones and their importance to women.

Q. What are the female sex hormones?

A. The two principal types of female sex hormones are estrogen and progesterone. The term estrogen usually is used in the singular, but there are in fact three major types of estrogen (plus many minor variations). The estrogens are made mostly in the ovaries, but many other tissues, such as fat and even skin, can also make estrogen. Progesterone is also is made mostly in the ovaries.

These two types of hormones are very important to a woman's reproductive functions. In young girls, estrogen is responsible for growing the sexually distinctive tissues, such as the vagina, uterus, ovaries, and breasts. Once a woman reaches sexual maturity, estrogen is important in maintaining the normal functioning of those tissues. We know far less about progesterone, although it often is referred to as the "pregnancy hormone" because it plays an important role in maintaining pregnancy. In nonpregnant woman, progesterone helps counterbalance some of the effects of estrogen, such as its growth-promoting effect on the uterus.

Q. Why is estrogen so important to my body?

A. At one time, doctors and scientists thought that the only purpose estrogen had in the body was to maintain the functioning of the female reproductive tissues. That theory was discarded after it was discovered that men also made estrogen, though in very small amounts.

We now know that estrogens play a role in the functioning of virtually every tissue in the body. Their ability to stimulate the growth of cells in reproductive tissues like the breast and the uterus remains their major role, but they also have a wide range of other beneficial effects not associated with reproduction, including:

- Stimulating the growth of bone cells
- Relaxing muscle cells in arteries and thereby lowing blood pressure
- Helping skin retain water and maintaining normal collagen, so it stays smooth and wrinkle free
- Reducing levels of the "bad," or low-density lipoprotein (LDL), form of cholesterol
- Increasing muscle energy levels
- Increasing short-term memory

When a woman has adequate levels of estrogen, it is quite apparent both to herself and to those around her that her skin is smooth and moist, her hair is lustrous and shiny, her disposition is confident and happy, and she has plenty of energy and strong muscle tone. Women who are said to "bloom" in appearance and disposition during pregnancy do so largely because estrogen levels rise to very high levels during pregnancy.

Q. Do I stop making estrogen completely when I become menopausal?

A. It is important to understand that once you enter menopause, your body doesn't stop making estrogen. It is just that it doesn't make as much as when you were younger. The ovaries continue making small amounts of estrogen and progesterone for the rest of a woman's life. Interestingly, however, the body now calls on its reserves to assist the ovaries; a wide range of tissues as diverse as the adrenal glands, brain, fat, muscle, skin, and gut wall also make these sex hormones. Collectively, however, these tissues only produce about 10 percent of the amount that was made in your body before menopause.

Q. What is the effect of low estrogen levels on my body during menopause?

A. The end result of lower estrogen levels is to reduce the nourishing effect of the hormone on all of the body's parts. Without high levels of this "youthful" hormone, tissues start to age at an accelerated rate. We'll look at the symptoms of menopause in greater detail in the next chapter, but for now, let's summarize the effects of falling estrogen levels as follows: The skin and lining of the vagina become drier and thinner, the bones become less resilient, the brain starts to lose its capacity for concentration and memory, muscle tone diminishes, energy levels start to fall, cataracts start to form, blood pressure rises, and blood vessels become more prone to damage from oxidized cholesterol and clotting. Even though a variety of tissues are making estrogen, the reality is that they are unable to make as much estrogen as they need to maintain the body's former vigor and youthfulness. Later in this book, we'll be looking at how the phytoestrogens provide a natural additional supply of estrogens to help keep tissues invigorated.

Q. How important is progesterone to me in menopause?

A. One of the main functions of progesterone in the menopausal woman is to act as a "pro-hormone" for estrogen. This term simply means that the body has to make progesterone before it can make estrogen. In an individual cell, for example a cell in the ovary, the manufacturing process of estrogen starts with a molecule of cholesterol. The cholesterol is converted by the cell's chemical factory into progesterone, and the progesterone molecule then is converted into estrogen. In the younger woman, at least 90 percent of all progesterone made in the body is eventually converted into other hormones, such as estrogen. Any progesterone that isn't converted to estrogen is used by the body for purposes such as helping to maintain pregnancy and to reverse the effects of estrogen on the lining of the uterus each month to result in menstruation.

Q. Why do I make testosterone?

A. Women make a surprisingly large amount of testosterone throughout life and the levels of testosterone don't fall after menopause quite as much as estrogen levels do. Testosterone is important to women in a couple of ways. Firstly, it is important in stimulating libido (sexual urge). Secondly, it is responsible for hair growth.

3.

The Effects of Menopause

Every woman can expect to experience some change as a result of a falling level of estrogen. It is too important a hormone and too broadly acting not to be missed when its levels decline by 80 to 90 percent during menopause. However, while some women feel that their bodies and minds have been significantly disrupted by the change, in other women the change may be hardly noticeable. In this chapter, we'll look at some of the changes most women can expect and mention a few ways to deal with or alleviate specific symptoms.

Q. What are the effects of menopause on my reproductive tissues?

A. Estrogen is so vital to the maintenance of the reproductive tissues that menopause brings about significant changes to their appearances as well as to their functions. There are three principal physical changes.

Firstly, the uterus shrinks. Without estrogen to stimulate the growth of the uterus, it becomes considerably smaller in menopausal woman.

Secondly, the vagina becomes drier, thinner, and less elastic. One of the important effects of estrogen is to keep the lining of the vagina moist and well lubricated. Menopausal women often find that intercourse becomes painful.

Thirdly, the breasts shrink. Estrogens promote growth of the glandular cells in the breasts. In menopause, these glandular cells virtually disappear and leave behind mostly fat. As a result, breasts normally shrink and become less firm. Women who have suffered painful PMS symptoms, such as cystic breast disease, normally find that their symptoms disappear with the onset of menopause.

Q. Is there any treatment for vaginal dryness?

A. Vaginal dryness can be one of the more uncomfortable side effects of menopause. Many women report finding intercourse painful after menopause, to the point that they lose their urge to have sex. Vaginal atrophy (thinning of the vagina) and dryness are usually easily managed by the use of lubricants in intercourse or by the application of local estrogen creams that quickly restore the vagina to a more youthful state in most cases. Also, strange though it may sound, more frequent intercourse reduces vaginal dryness overall.

A dry vagina is also predisposed to yeast infection (*Candida albicans*). Anti-fungal creams prescribed by a doctor are normally very effective. Some holistic physicians recommend *Lactobacillus acidophilus* supplements or yogurt for this problem, particularly if antibiotics have diminished the amount of helpful *Lactobacillus acidophilus* in the gut, which can lead to an overgrowth of *Candida*. As for yogurt, you need to read labels to be sure that there are sufficient amounts of *Lactobacillus acidophilus* present.

Q. What are the effects on other parts of my body?

A. The sorts of effects discussed above on reproductive tissues generally are accepted and understood by women as being a normal and inevitable part of menopause. However, there are a range of other effects that are not so well understood. For example, many don't understand why they feel bad-tempered, want to cry over trivial things, feel lethargic, or are not able to control their urine. These are all consequences of low or falling levels of estrogen. Some symptoms are associated with peri-menopause while others are the consequences of menopause.

Perimenopause is really the start of menopause. The symptoms at this time are those associated with falling estrogen levels. The main perimenopausal effects are hot flashes, night sweats, and mood swings.

Post-menopause is when estrogen levels have stopped falling and have leveled out. The effects at this time are associated with long-term low estrogen levels. The main post-menopausal effects are joint aches, incontinence, osteoporosis, atherosclerosis, high blood pressure, cataract formation, muscle weakness, and general feelings of fatigue.

Q. What are hot flashes?

A. Some 80 percent of women in Western countries report that they experience hot flashes during menopause. A hot flash is exactly as the term suggests—a feeling of being overheated that comes and goes, more or less, in a flash. Hot flashes aren't always so quick, however. Each hot flash can last from several minutes to about an hour, and a woman can experience from one to more than forty episodes a day. They can occur day or night, and can be severe enough at night to awaken a woman. When they occur at night, they're called night sweats.

No one is absolutely sure what causes a hot flash, although it seems to be associated with sudden estrogen withdrawal because men coming off estrogen therapy for prostatic disease also experience hot flashes. It may result from a malfunction within the part of the brain responsible for regulating body heat.

Q. Does anything help ease hot flashes and night sweats?

A. Many women can minimize the effects of hot flashes through commonsense measures, such as dressing in light layers that can be removed or added as the need arises. A small hand fan can be used to cool the face. A cool or tepid (not hot) shower before going to bed may help prevent or minimize hot flashes and night sweats. Wearing light nightclothes, using thin cotton or wool blankets, and sleeping in a cool room can help. Doctors often recommend avoiding caffeine or alcohol before going to bed. Stress can lead to hot flashes, so relaxation techniques, such as deep-breathing exercises and meditation, may be helpful.

If hot flashes are caused by the sudden withdrawal of estrogen, it would appear that anything that results in a slowed rate of withdrawal should help. Providing the body with additional estrogen may help. Later in this book, we look at phytoestrogens as a source for regulation of the body's estrogen levels.

Q. What is osteoporosis?

A. Osteoporosis refers to progressive thinning and weakening of the bones—to the point that they cannot support the weight of the body. Most fractures in men and women over the age of forty-five are due to osteoporosis, and it is responsible for an estimated 1.3 million fractures in the United States annually at a cost of $10 billion. Elderly women are seven times more likely to experience a fracture than elderly men.

Osteoporosis also leads to compression in the vertebrae of our backs because they get softer. This is one reason we get shorter as we age. In severe cases, it can also lead to curvature of the spine and formation of the classic "dowager's hump" in the upper part of the spine.

We tend to think of our bones as inert, solid masses. In fact, however, bone is living tissue, and like all living tissue, it is in a constant state of flux. Bone tissue is constantly broken down and replaced with new tissue, and estrogens play an important part in this remodeling process. Bone tissue contains two particular types of cells known as osteoclasts and osteoblasts. The osteoclasts break down the bone tissue while the osteoblasts lay down new bone tissue. These two types of cells are working constantly in concert in order to keep the bones healthy.

When we are young and growing, there is more bone growth than bone removal. Between the ages of about twenty and forty-five, the two opposite functions are held in equilibrium, so our bones are neither gaining nor losing density. However, from middle age onward, the balance shifts towards losing; bone is being removed at a faster rate than it is replaced. The osteoclasts (the destroyers) are working harder than the osteoblasts (the builders) during this time of life. Osteoporosis simply refers to this aging process whereby our bones become thinner. Osteoporosis starts being a serious problem when our bones get so weak that they fracture easily when we bump into things. Even the simple act of sneezing or coughing can lead to fractures of ribs if osteoporosis is sufficiently bad.

Q. Why is osteoporosis associated with menopause?

A. Osteoporosis occurs in menopausal women because of low estrogen levels. Following menopause, a woman's bone density falls at a rate of 1 to 3 percent per year. Estrogen has a major influence on the balance between bone construction and bone breakdown. It stimulates the cells responsible for building bone and inhibits the cells responsible for destroying bone. Estrogen also appears to assist in the absorption of calcium from the diet.

Q. Will diet help me reduce the risk of osteoporosis?

A. You cannot completely prevent osteoporosis because it is a natural part of aging. You can, however, prevent the rate at which it occurs and probably prevent it from getting so bad that you are at risk of a fracture if you fall.

One of the important things to do is to make sure that you have good levels in the diet of the main building blocks of bone: calcium, magnesium, and vitamin D. These are found naturally in foods and are also available as mineral and vitamin supplements. Fresh fruits and vegetables, particularly cabbage, broccoli, and cauliflower, along with dairy products (milk, cheese, and yogurt), are good natural sources of these important building blocks.

Recent research also suggests that vitamin C is important in the fight against osteoporosis. Vitamin C is necessary for the activity of an important enzyme used in the synthesis of collagen, a major component of bone. According to Melvyn Werbach, M.D., while the possibility that vitamin C deficiency contributes to osteoporosis has not been proved, vitamin C supplementation is generally so safe that it seems worthwhile to take to prevent this possible problem.

Caffeine has been shown to interfere with the absorption of calcium from the diet; tea and coffee, therefore, should be used in moderation. Recent studies, however, have found that one glass of milk per day can offset the deleterious effects of caffeine on calcium absorption.

Q. What else can I do to prevent osteoporosis?

A. The importance of exercise can hardly be over-emphasized in osteoporosis prevention. Exercise stimulates the growth of new bone cells. Again, we will also be looking later on at phytoestrogens, which may help prove helpful in countering osteoporosis.

Q. How does cardiovascular disease affect menopausal women?

A. Cardiovascular diseases, such as coronary artery disease and strokes, are the most common diseases in menopausal women. They account for about half of all deaths of women in Western countries. At the age of forty, women have about one-third of the risk of having a heart attack that men of the same age have. After menopause, however, women begin to lose this privileged status. By the age of seventy-five, a woman has the same risk of heart attack or stroke as a man of the same age. The main reason seems to be the loss of estrogen's protective effect on the cardiovascular system. Younger women are relatively protected because of their high estrogen levels, and this protective effect is lost with menopause.

Following menopause, a number of changes may take place in a woman's blood vessels. The most important potential development is a condition known as atherosclerosis, which is characterized by fatty deposits on the lining of the arteries. Atherosclerosis is associated with cholesterol. Present in our bodies are two main forms of cholesterol: low density lipoprotein (LDL) cholesterol, which is the "bad" kind, and high density lipoprotein (HDL) cholesterol, which is the "good" kind. LDL cholesterol predisposes us to atherosclerosis while HDL cholesterol provides protection against this condition. A healthy cholesterol profile is one where the LDL cholesterol level is not much higher than the HDL cholesterol level. When this is the case, HDL cholesterol is able to prevent LDL cholesterol from attaching to artery walls. However, if LDL cholesterol levels rise, there arises a buildup of cholesterol in the lining of the arteries.

The next stage of the process of atherosclerosis is when the cholesterol in the artery walls becomes oxidized by molecules known as free radicals. Oxidized cholesterol becomes toxic to the surrounding tissue and results in an inflammation in the lining of the arteries and also causes blood to clot. The combined effect of these two events closes off the artery and prevents any blood from getting through. This can happen to arteries all over the body, but the consequences of its happening in some arteries can be worse than its happening in others. For example, if the arteries supplying the heart muscle (coronary arteries) get blocked, then the end result is usually a heart attack. If the carotid artery (the main artery supplying the head) is affected, then the end result may be a stroke.

High estrogen levels are associated with a low risk of developing coronary heart disease in women. The hormone provides a number of important beneficial effects for the cardiovascular system, and its absence in this capacity is often very apparent.

Estrogen is a very good cholesterol-lowering agent. The prescription medications that are currently available to lower cholesterol act by reducing LDL levels but have little or no effect on HDL levels. Estrogen, on the other hand, pushes up HDL levels while at the same time lowering LDL levels. This dual effect is thought to be more beneficial in terms of preventing atherosclerosis. Estrogen does this by instructing the liver to convert LDL cholesterol to HDL cholesterol. Menopausal women are deprived of this beneficial effect, thereby leading to a lower HDL to LDL cholesterol ratio and a higher overall cholesterol level.

Estrogen is also an antioxidant, which means that it helps prevent the oxidation of any LDL cholesterol that does manage to lodge in the arteries. In menopausal women, lower estrogen levels mean that LDL cholesterol is more prone to oxidation.

Estrogen also has anti-inflammatory properties,

which means that it helps control the inflammations that build up in the artery walls in response to oxidation of LDL cholesterol.

Q. What can I do to reduce the risk of cardiovascular disease after menopause?

A. You can reduce the risk of cardiovascular disease by taking several important steps. Firstly, eat a sensible diet containing low levels of saturated fats (a major source of LDL cholesterol) and significant quantities of fruits and vegetables containing antioxidant vitamins to help prevent cholesterol oxidation. Secondly, maintain a reasonable weight. Thirdly, exercise regularly. Even a daily walk can help keep the heart and arteries fit. Fourthly, avoid tobacco and exposure to tobacco (second-hand smoke). Fifthly, learn ways to deal with or avoid stress. Lastly, a natural phytoestrogen supplement may help offset the estrogen loss of menopause.

Although these steps probably will not completely overcome the adverse consequences of low estrogen levels, they are sensible steps that can and should be taken to reduce the impact of menopause on the cardiovascular system.

Q. What causes general aches and pains?

A. One of the actions of estrogen is to help keep the connective tissue in the body supple and flexible. Connective tissue, which is composed largely of a protein called collagen, helps provide the support structure of the body as ligaments and tendons. When estrogen levels fall, this structure becomes stiffer, which results in general aches and pains in joints and the back. This loss of collagen flexibility is also one of the main reasons that skin becomes more wrinkled in menopausal women.

Q. Why do menopausal women sometimes have bladder problems?

A. This has to do with the action of estrogen on muscles. Estrogen helps muscles keep their tone and strength, and one of the important muscles affected by estrogen in this way is the small sphincter muscle around the neck of the bladder. Normally, the sphincter muscle is contracted, which keeps the bladder closed. When a woman wants to pass urine, this muscle relaxes and allows urine to pass out of the bladder. Estrogen plays an important part in helping this muscle stay contracted. Consequently, in menopausal women the muscle tends to relax, which makes it difficult to retain urine. Sometimes, the result is incontinence.

4.

How to Manage Menopause

From here on, we're going to concentrate on the options available to woman to effectively manage estrogen-related health issues. There are no hard and fast rules; the statement that every woman should be on a hormone replacement therapy (HRT) of some kind is just as wrong as saying that alternatives to HRT are the way to go for every woman. Each woman is the best judge of what she needs, and making an informed decision requires that a woman understand the different options available to her.

Q. Doesn't menopause effectively signal the end of the productive part of a woman's life?

A. It does not at all. Most women will live another thirty years after the beginning of menopause, and these should be some of the most rewarding years of her life. Usually having raised her children already, she can devote time and energy to hobbies, travel, education, and friends.

The best advice that can be offered to a woman facing menopause is to adopt a positive outlook and to regard menopause as a time of freedom and opportunity. It is a good time to take stock of one's life and determine what is to be accomplished in the many years ahead.

Q. If menopause is natural, why do American women suffer so much?

A. The fact that so many American women suffer from hot flashes in their perimenopausal years and cardiovascular disease and osteoporosis in their later years has led to the notion that menopause is an "estrogen-deficiency" disease that needs to be treated aggressively with synthetic estrogens. However, there is an alternative view that says that this suffering is not natural and is largely avoidable. This holistic approach to menopause is summarized in three sequential, logical conclusions.

Firstly, menopause is a natural event. Nature has sound biological reasons for leading a woman into menopause.

Secondly, as a natural event, it is not likely to be life-damaging or life-threatening, particularly for a period that is one-third of a woman's life.

Thirdly, if severe menopausal symptoms are not natural, then there must be something in the lifestyle of the modern woman that is predisposing her to suffer such symptoms. That something is a typical American diet low in natural phytoestrogens that would alleviate many menopausal symptoms.

Q. Do women all over the world have the same problem with menopause?

A. No, and this single fact is the very basis of this book. We know that the symptoms of estrogen deficiency observed in menopausal women in the United States and other Western countries don't seem to be prevalent elsewhere. This applies to both perimenopausal symptoms (such as hot flashes) and post-menopausal symptoms (such as incontinence, bone fractures, and heart disease). Throughout Asian countries (such as Malaysia, Indonesia, Thailand, China, and Japan), the Indian subcontinent, the Middle East, and South America, symptoms of menopause are not particularly dramatic. Women of those countries do not seem to need the medical attention that their American counterparts do because the symptoms either don't exist or are not severe enough to warrant medical help. Initially, it was thought that this was perhaps just a cultural difference, that women in such areas were not encouraged to speak of their symptoms, or that perhaps the very business of living and surviving overrode any "self-pity." However, there is evidence that this is not the case.

Q. What are some differences between the menopausal symptoms of Western women and the symptoms of women from other parts of the world?

A. A study of Japanese menopausal women, carried out by Dr. Margaret Lock and described in the journals *Maturitas* and *Experimental Gerontology*, found that only 9 percent of these women reported hot flashes and only 3 percent reported night sweats. To her amazement, Lock found that hot flashes were so infrequent and unbothersome that the Japanese language has no term for "hot flash." Lock also noted, "Every Japanese doctor interviewed during the survey and since that time confirms that hot flashes are not symptoms about which Japanese women consult a doctor." This compares with a reported rate of about 80 percent of American women who experience hot flashes to the extent that they consult a doctor. The most common symptoms reported in the study were stiff shoulders (52 percent) and headaches (22 percent).

The longer-term outlook also is much different for menopausal Japanese women, with the rates of osteoporosis and fractures of the hip being only half of those of U.S. women of equivalent age. The death rate from heart disease of Japanese women is only about one-quarter of that of U.S. women.

Researchers have found similar patterns in other countries where people have diets different from the typical Western diet. For example, Thai researchers reported that only 3 percent of menopausal women were completely free of symptoms but that their symptoms were very different from those experienced by Western women. The most common symptoms experienced by Thai women in the survey were backaches (26 percent), headaches (25 percent), dizziness (25 percent), forgetfulness (24 percent), and joint pains (23 percent). Overall, these symptoms were mild in intensity. The more dramatic "American" symptoms of hot flashes (16 percent), night sweats (9 percent), and incontinence (10 percent) ranked quite low on the list of symptoms afflicting Thai women.

In South America as well, native Mayan women have no concept of hot flashes and, like the Japanese and Chinese, have no word for this symptom.

Q. What protects these women from menopausal symptoms?

A. While women in traditional societies don't entirely escape the effects of menopause, they don't suffer the same symptoms that American women do. It is almost as if they were experiencing mild effects of a changing hormonal composition. It seems little worse than the effects that woman experience when they go through puberty and their sex-hormone levels are changing.

There are almost certainly a whole range of lifestyle factors protecting women from traditional societies from the adverse effects of menopause. One factor stands out above all others: the fact that the diets of most traditionally living people are high in natural plant estrogens. The typical Western diet, by contrast, has very low levels of these plant compounds.

We now know that plant estrogens can perform many of the functions of a woman's steroidal estrogens. Although plant estrogens are much weaker than the estrogens produced by the ovaries, they

can be present in the body at levels ma⟋
of times greater than steroidal estrogen
ple, Japanese researchers found that individuals
who consumed a typical Japanese diet had levels of
plant estrogens in their bodies of up to 10,000 times
that of their steroidal estrogens. These plant estrogens were coming from legumes such as soy, a sta-
ple of the Japanese diet.

Q. What about women in areas such as Mexico and India who aren't eating soy? Where do they obtain their phytoestrogens?

A. What all of these women, the Japanese as well
as the Mexican and Indian, have in common is that
they eat a type of vegetable known as a legume. In
Japan, the main legume eaten is soy; in Mexico,
India, and other parts of the world, the main
legumes eaten are chickpeas, lentils, and beans. All
of these legumes are a rich source of phytoestrogens.

Many researchers now believe that plant estrogens hold the key to the riddle of the lower inci-
dences of menopausal symptoms in different cultures around the world as compared with those of

Western countries. Plant estrogens provide a supplementary source of estrogens, which helps to soften the onset of menopause and forestalls many short-term problems, such as hot flashes and mood swings. These plant estrogens also support a woman's body during her life after menopause and prevent some long-term problems, such as heart disease and osteoporosis.

Q. Do I need to take hormone replacement therapy (HRT)?

A. That is for you and your physician to decide. However, considering the many side effects associated with synthetic estrogen and the sort of alternatives provided in this book, more doctors are viewing hormone replacement therapy as a last resort. There is no doubt that the agent used in HRT is a powerful drug; however, therein lies the problem— it is a drug. To many women, it seems bizarre that they should be taking a drug for possibly the rest of their lives.

A 1994 Gallup Poll showed that 40 percent of menopausal women in the United States have used HRT (with estrogen alone or in combination with progesterone). HRT is mostly used in the short term to control the acute symptoms of perimenopause, especially hot flashes. For these women, the use of HRT to relieve menopausal symptoms can be a blessing. Increasingly, though, under the influence of more aggressive drug company advertising, doctors are recommending that their patients consider taking HRT on a long-term basis to counteract the adverse consequences of long-term low estrogen levels, such as osteoporosis and cardiovascular disease. Now the prospect of using estrogens for twenty to thirty years with all of their attendant side effects to gain some health benefits is a decision that is going to face more and more women. As a prominent gynecologist at Massachusetts General Hospital said recently, "Basically, you're presenting women with the possibility of increasing the risk of getting breast cancer at age sixty in order to prevent a heart attack at age seventy and a hip fracture at age eighty. How can you make that decision for a patient?"

Q. Is there a difference in the thought behind the HRT and holistic approaches?

A. The HRT approach stems from the view that menopause is a medical condition and that, through some accident of nature, women are exposed in later life to a hormone deficiency. The holistic argument, on the other hand, is that a low estrogen level in later life is not a biological mistake. The proponents of this view argue that it makes little sense to put potent hormones back into the body when nature has it present in low levels.

Proponents of a holistic approach would also point out that doctors use hormones to treat hormone-deficiency disorders, as growth hormone is used to treat dwarfism. Menopause is not a disease state or disorder (as dwarfism is) and a low estrogen level is not an abnormality. To add hormones to a natural state is to invite problems.

Q. Why is HRT so frequently recommended by doctors?

A. The 1960s book *Feminine Forever*, by Robert Wilson, M.D., conditioned some people to think that menopause is a hormone deficiency state that requires drug treatment. This notion led to the idea that replacement estrogen therapy is the lifeblood of the menopausal woman and that virtually every woman over the age of fifty was depriving herself of the benefits of a healthy older age if she failed to take steroidal hormones.

This medication of menopause continues today as part of mainstream medicine. Take, for example, a quotation attributed to Dr. Theresa Crenshaw in *The Philadelphia Inquirer* that menopause "is not a natural condition, it is an endocrine disorder and should be treated medically with the same seriousness we treat other endocrine disorders, such as diabetes or thyroid disease."

It must be said, however, that HRT does work. For a woman suffering severe hot flashes and night sweats, HRT can be a tremendous relief. It usually provides relief from these symptoms within a week or two of starting treatment. Over the long term, though, there is an increased risk of breast and endometrial cancers with HRT.

Q. Why do so many women stop taking HRT?

A. A number of surveys carried out in different countries, including the United States, have shown that most women who start HRT fail to complete the prescribed course. The main reason for this is a high rate of side effects. These side effects include headaches, nausea, liver disorders, fluid retention (which causes bloating), depression, breakthrough bleeding, endometrial hypertrophy, enlargement of uterine fibroids, breast tenderness, increased risk of gallstones, and weight gain (averaging eight pounds). These are some of the more minor or non-life-threatening side effects. On a more serious note, there is an increased risk of blood clot formation, breast cancer, and other cancers.

The female sex hormone system is so intricate, complex, and finely balanced that to think that it is possible to readjust the system by adding one or two hormones is very simplistic. In light of this, the option of supplementation with a natural phyto-estrogen is one well worth considering.

5.

Phytoestrogens and Isoflavones

Phytoestrogens provide a significant level of estrogenic activity for the body. These estrogens, from plants such as red clover, possess many of the beneficial properties of actual hormones without, apparently, any of the side effects. In this chapter, we look at phytoestrogens and narrow in on some of the most beneficial plant estrogens—the isoflavones.

Q. Why do phytoestrogens work as estrogens in the body?

A. In order for human estrogen to have an effect on the body, it must be received by individual cells; the cell's "estrogen receptor" is what allows the cell to respond to estrogen. Because of the chemical similarity between human estrogens and phytoestrogens, the cell's estrogen receptor will also respond to phytoestrogens. Though the cell's receptor is less responsive to plant estrogen than it is to human estrogen or the estrogens used in HRT, the difference is somewhat offset by the huge number of phytoestrogens that can be supplied by the diet or a supplement and carried by the bloodstream.

Q. Is there only one type of phytoestrogen?

A. No, there are many different types. They all are drawn from the same chemical family known as phenolics, which are the largest chemical group in plants (with over 4,000 different types known). From this large family of compounds, we presently know of eighteen that are estrogenic in humans; these are the ones that we call phytoestrogens. In time, scientists likely will discover that additional phenolics have estrogen-like properties.

We can divide these eighteen phenolic phytoestrogens further into seven different subgroups based on chemical structure: flavanones, flavones, flavanols, isoflavones, coumestans, lignans, and chalcones. Isoflavones and coumestans are the most estrogenic; they are about ten times stronger than the others.

Q. What sorts of plants contain phytoestrogens?

A. Phytoestrogens are present in all plants. Every single vegetable, fruit, or cereal that we eat has at least one type of phytoestrogen present. The flavones and flavonols are mostly red- and yellow-colored pigments and are found in colored fruits and vegetables. Red grapes, and so red wines, are a good source of estrogenic flavones. Flavanones are restricted largely to citrus fruits, such as grapefruit and oranges. Lignans are found virtually in all fruits, vegetables, and cereals, but linseed is the richest source of estrogenic lignans. Estrogenic isoflavones and coumestans are found almost solely in vegetables known as legumes.

Q. How much phytoestrogen am I likely to get in my diet?

A. The answer depends on how many fruit and vegetables you are eating and what types you are eating. It has been estimated that the average American eats between 50 and 200 mg of phytoestrogens each day and that most of these are flavones and flavonols (fruits), flavanones (citrus fruit juice), and lignans (cereals and most fruits and vegetables). There is probably no more than from 1 to 3 mg of estrogenic isoflavones per day in the typical American diet.

A vegetarian diet obviously gives a much higher phytoestrogen level, probably two to three times the average level, because of the greater amount of plant material consumed. More importantly, the types of phytoestrogens present in the vegetarian, Latin-American, or Asian diet will be different. Legume-eating people obtain good amounts of estrogenic isoflavones (between 10 and 100+ mg a day).

Q. Are herbs a good source of phytoestrogens?

A. Herbs, being plants, obviously contain a certain level of phytoestrogens. Some herbs in particular are known to contain relatively potent phytoestrogens. The problem is that in general very little is known about the nature of the phytoestrogens present. The experience with an herbal plant grown in Thailand should serve as a caution about other herbs used for estrogenic effects. This particular plant has been used for centuries in Thailand by some communities for its estrogenic effects. A recent study identified the active component as a compound called miroestrol. Unlike the main kinds of phytoestrogens that we have been talking about that have a phenolic chemical structure, miroestrol is a steroidal estrogen. That is, it is part of the same chemical family as the estrogens made in the body and is fairly potent. Eating this herb, in fact, is little different from taking HRT.

Q. What exactly are isoflavones?

A. Isoflavones are the most important type of phytoestrogen found in the human diet. All of the different types of phytoestrogens that we eat every day undoubtedly contribute in some way to health, but it is the high potency of the isoflavones and their range of biological effects that suggest that they contribute the most. Ironically, isoflavones are the one type of phytoestrogen that most women in America and other Western countries are lacking in their diets.

Out of the 1,000 or so different isoflavones found in plants, four have been shown to be estrogenic and of particular importance to humans. These are:

- Genistein
- Biochanin
- Daidzein
- Formononetin

Although these terms may be very unfamiliar, they are very important. You'll be learning more about them shortly. For now, just remember that every time that you eat a legume, you are going to eat at least one of these four estrogenic isoflavones.

By the way, don't worry about men eating these isoflavones in legumes. There is research showing that they also deliver many health benefits to men. For example, they may reduce the risk of prostate cancer.

Q. What health benefits do isoflavones have for the body, and how do they work?

A. One of the main effects in the body of all the different phytoestrogens is their ability to mimic estrogens. The four key estrogenic isoflavones look so much like estrogens to the cell that they are able to "trick" cells into responding to them. They are not as nearly as potent as estradiol, the strongest of the estrogens, but a high-legume diet delivers such a high level of estrogenic isoflavones to the blood, that their overall estrogenic effect is quite powerful. The estrogenic health benefits from these isoflavones include, at least in some degree, all of those attributed to estrogens.

Q. Do isoflavones behave just like human estrogens?

A. Estradiol (either naturally occurring or that used in HRT) is entirely nonselective as to which cells it stimulates. It attaches as easily to the estrogen receptors in every tissue of the body. This is why the estradiol in HRT produces a mixture of good and bad effects in the menopausal woman. Activating cells in the bone, heart, and brain, for example, is desirable, but activating cells in the breast and the uterus is often undesirable (especially at a certain age) and can result in breast tenderness, uterine bleeding, and cancers of both tissues.

In contrast, isoflavones show little inclination to attach to breast and uterine cells. They do, however, attach quite strongly to cells in bone, the heart, and the brain. This means that they can provide positive estrogenic effects for the body without causing the unwanted side effects normally associated with HRT. On the other hand, the fact that isoflavones don't stimulate the lining of the reproductive tract means that they won't do much to relieve vaginal atrophy. This problem, however, is easily dealt with by the use of lubricants or a local estrogen cream.

Q. Is it true that isoflavones also have anti-cancer properties?

A. A large number of laboratory studies have suggested that isoflavones have potent anti-cancer qualities. In these test-tube studies, each of the four estrogenic isoflavones has been shown to suppress the growth of cells of human breast cancer, prostate cancer, bowel cancer, and leukemia. While promising, this research is far from confirming that isoflavones can prevent cancer or be an effective treatment in people with cancer.

Laboratory studies also seem to suggest that isoflavones can prompt some cancer cells to revert back to normal cells and then die naturally. This is accomplished by turning on the "switch" that instructs cells to die after a certain time, which cancer cells manage to turn off. However, the action of an isoflavone turning on this switch in cancerous human tissue has only been observed in a laboratory, not in a person.

Isoflavones appear to prevent cancers in another important way: They prevent the growth of new blood vessels. This is called angiogenic inhibition. By depriving fast-growing tumors of a vital blood supply, it has been shown that the spread of cancer can be prevented. The discovery of this anti-cancer property of isoflavones is exciting and merits further scientific research.

In the *Lancet* in 1997, Dr. David Ingram, a breast cancer surgeon, reported that the risk of getting breast cancer was lowered when isoflavone levels in the body were very high. He took a group of several hundred Australian women who were all considered to be at a high risk of breast cancer because of a family history of breast cancer. He divided these women into those who had developed breast cancer and those who had not, and he found that levels of isoflavones in the urine (reflecting dietary intake) was significantly greater in the group that hadn't developed breast cancer than in those women who had developed breast cancer.

Q. Is there one isoflavone that seems to have greater anti-cancer properties than the others?

A. Many studies have focused on genistein as a potential anti-cancer agent, and genistein does have good anti-cancer properties in the test tube. However, it is far from being the most important in terms of anti-cancer action. For example, recent research has shown that daidzein and formononetin are converted in the body into compounds that actually are more potent anti-cancer agents than genistein. Also, biochanin has been shown in some laboratory studies to be a more effective agent than genistein against human breast cancer cells.

Q. What other effects do isoflavones have on the body?

A. Isoflavones are turning out to be quite remarkable plant compounds. We have probably only scratched the surface of understanding the full implications of isoflavones for human health. In addition to their estrogenic and anti-cancer effects, they also are diuretics, have anti-inflammatory properties, can stimulate the immune system, and are potent antioxidants.

Q. How much of isoflavones do I need each day?

A. Although no one knows what the ideal dose is for women, we do have some general ideas from studies conducted that have seen health benefits of isoflavones in cultures in which legumes are prevalent. The daily dietary intake of these four main isoflavones in Japan and China can range between about 15 and 100 mg. The more usual range quoted by researchers for traditional cultures like Japan is 30 to 40 mg per day. It therefore seems that people should aim for about 40 mg per day.

Q. How do I get isoflavones?

A. The only way to get them through the diet is to eat legumes, that is, by consuming plants such as red clover, chick peas (found in hummus), soy (soybeans, soy milk products, and tofu), lentils, and various kinds of beans (mung beans, lima beans, haricot beans, navy beans, etc.). Like the levels of any nutrient, the levels of the four estrogenic isoflavones in these foods will vary greatly. Taking soy as an example, the isoflavone levels will vary considerably depending on the variety of bean, where and how the beans were grown and stored, and how they were processed. Some soy milks have virtually no isoflavones present, so it is important to be aware of possible differences. Alternatively, you can take a dietary supplement rich with isoflavones that is derived from legumes.

Q. Why are isoflavones present in legumes?

A. The reason relates to the nature of legumes. Legumes are especially efficient in taking nitrogen from the air and soil and converting it into protein. (For this reason, legumes have higher levels of protein than other plants, which is why so many cultures use legumes as a good dietary source of protein.) The legume accomplishes this conversion of nitrogen to protein with the help of soil-dwelling bacteria. Isoflavones play a key role in this process— they are the bait for this bacteria. Legumes must keep a good supply of isoflavones on hand to attract the bacteria necessary for its protein production.

Q. Do I need to get all four estrogenic isoflavones in my diet?

A. The answer appears to be yes. Each of the four estrogenic isoflavones has its own biological characteristics. It is not possible to point to any one isoflavone as being the most important; each is quite different in its estrogenic, anti-cancer, and antioxidant properties. Since most women want a full range of health benefits, all four isoflavones should be present in the diet. All of the current evidence suggests that the four major isoflavones act independently and in a complementary manner.

Genistein is a moderate estrogen and anti-cancer agent, and is a weak antioxidant.

Biochanin is a weaker estrogen than genistein (about one-tenth as estrogenic), but is a more effective anti-cancer agent in some situations. A number of studies have shown that biochanin is more effective than genistein in protecting human breast cancer cells against the proliferative effects of estradiol. If human breast cancer cells are put in a test tube and observed, they show a slow and steady multiplication. If estradiol is added, the rate of multiplication speeds up dramatically. Adding biochanin to the mix instead of estradiol is far more effective than adding genistein in blocking the stimulatory effect of estradiol on the cancer cells. Some of the biochanin that we eat is converted in the body into genistein, but about one-third remains as biochanin and, therefore, has its own impact on the body.

Daidzein is less estrogenic than genistein (about one-tenth as strong) and has virtually no anti-cancer effect. However, it is a potent antioxidant. Also, daidzein is converted in the body into different end-products, many of which are more estrogenic and have greater anti-cancer properties than genistein.

Formononetin is a weak isoflavone in that it has

weak estrogenic, anti-cancer, and antioxidant properties. However, almost all of the formononetin that we eat is converted in the body into daidzein. The main function of formononetin in the diet is to provide a source of daidzein.

Q. Where do I find each of these four isoflavones in particular?

A. Genistein is distributed fairly widely in legumes (also known as pulses). It is the main isoflavone in soy and is also found in other pulses, such as lentils and some varieties of chickpeas.

Biochanin is the dominant isoflavone in clovers, chickpeas, and many varieties of lentils and beans widely used in South America. Chick peas that are freshly sprouted are an especially rich source of biochanin.

Daidzein is widely distributed in pulses, although its major sources are soy and kudzu (Japanese arrowroot).

Formononetin is the most commonly occurring of the four major estrogenic isoflavones. It is widely distributed in most legumes with the exception of soy and some varieties of chickpeas.

Most plants only have one or two of the four main estrogenic isoflavones. Soy, for example, only contains daidzein and genistein. Therefore, we often have to eat several different types of legumes to ensure that we have obtained all four. This is generally what happens because no society eats just one type of legume. For example, even though the Japanese eat a lot of soy products, they also eat other legumes, such as kudzu, mung beans, and lab-lab beans and, in so doing, obtain all four isoflavones.

Q. What happens to the isoflavones when they get into my body?

A. Isoflavones are readily absorbed from the diet into the body, but in the process they undergo a series of changes. The first change occurs when isoflavones reach the bowels. In its natural state, the isoflavone is attached to a sugar, such as glucose. The isoflavone in this form is referred to as a glycoside. In order for the isoflavone to be activated, it needs to be freed from its sugar. This happens in the gut by means of the bacteria present there. The bacteria use the sugar and in so doing they release the isoflavone. A high proportion of these liberated isoflavones then is absorbed across the gut wall into the bloodstream.

The second change occurs with the isoflavones that are absorbed. Genistein and daidzein undergo little further change, but biochanin and formononetin are most often modified by the liver. About half to two-thirds of the biochanin is converted to genistein, and about 90 percent of the formononetin is converted to daidzein.

Another change involves those isoflavones that were not absorbed immediately after being released from their sugar. These isoflavones are taken up by the bacteria in the gut and are fermented to produce a range of end-products called metabolites. All of these metabolites are absorbed into the bloodstream.

The effects from dietary isoflavones come from a combination of both the whole isoflavone and the isoflavone metabolite.

6.

The Red Clover Story

In this chapter we turn our attention at last to red clover. Very high levels of all four estrogenic isoflavones are to be found in red clover, which allows it to be easily processed into a convenient supplement. In both the short term and long term, red clover appears to be a very safe source of phytoestrogens for those who lack the time or the desire to eat legumes regularly.

Q. Why is red clover regarded as such a good source of isoflavones?

A. Most of the members of the clover family have high levels of isoflavones, although the common white clover has very low levels. Red clover, however, has very high levels—about 2 percent of the dry weight of its leaves is isoflavones. This is about ten times the isoflavone percentage in soy.

The other very important factor is the types of isoflavones present. Unlike other legumes, such as soy, which only contain daidzein and genistein, red clover contains all four main estrogenic isoflavones. The dominant isoflavones in red clover are biochanin and formononetin, but the body converts some of these two isoflavones into genistein and daidzein. Writing in a clinical monograph entitled *Standardized Extract of Red Clover*, Donald Brown, M.D. points out that red clover isoflavones given to people result in high blood levels of daidzein and genistein, moderate blood levels of biochanin, and low levels of formononetin. This is a similar profile to that seen in the blood of vegetarians who are eating a variety of legumes. In contrast, soy consumption does not result in any increase in biochanin or formononetin in the blood.

Why is red clover to be preferred to other sources of isoflavones? There are several reasons:

- It is the one plant that delivers all four major estrogenic isoflavones.
- Studies such as the aforementioned confirm that red clover isoflavones have estrogenic effects when consumed.
- Red clover's estrogenic isoflavone levels are very high, which means that it doesn't have to be concentrated too much in a dietary supplement.

- Red clover is generally considered to be a safe plant for human consumption.
- Red clover is not known to have any anti-nutritive factors (unlike soy) and is not known to cause allergies.

Q. What benefits does red clover offer menopausal women?

A. The first benefit is that it provides a convenient and safe way to obtain all four main estrogenic isoflavones without having to change your diet.

The second benefit is that the isoflavones in red clover provide an estrogenic effect as Dr. Brown mentioned on page 66. A red clover supplement, which supplies 40 mg of isoflavones per 500 mg tablet, was given to eighty-six perimenopausal women suffering from acute menopausal symptoms (such as hot flashes). The trials were double-blind and placebo-controlled, which means that half the women took a placebo (inactive) tablet and the other half an active (red-clover-isoflavones) tablet, and neither the women nor their doctors knew which tablet was which. The study continued for approximately eight months. Each week, the women recorded the frequency and severity of their hot flashes. A sample of their urine also was collected at the end of the study to determine how much of isoflavones was present in their bodies. The combined data showed that there was a very strong correlation between clinical response in the incidence of hot flashes and urinary levels of isoflavones. In other words, as isoflavones increased, hot flashes decreased. This was the first time that a direct health benefit of isoflavones was established in humans.

Q. Will red clover provide any long-term benefits?

A. Another apparent benefit of red clover is for the cardiovascular system. In a study reported by Professor John Eden, M.D., of the Royal Hospital for Women in Sydney, Australia, to the 1996 Meeting of the International Menopause Society, red clover treatment in menopausal women resulted in an average 18-percent rise in blood levels of HDL (or "good") cholesterol.

The isoflavones provided by red clover also have been reported to relax the artery walls of menopausal women, which is an effect likely to reduce the risk of high blood pressure. In a study by the eminent cardiovascular physician Paul Nestel, M.D., isoflavones yield a significant increase in the ability of the artery walls of menopausal women to relax.

Q. How were plant estrogens discovered?

A. The story began in the 1940s when researchers discovered a condition known as clover disease in sheep. In many parts of Australia, flocks of sheep were showing evidence of an oversupply of estrogen—the ewes simply stopped ovulating.

The problem was eventually traced to the large amounts of estrogenic isoflavones in their diet. It turned out that the animals were getting about one gram (1,000 mg) of estrogenic isoflavones in their diet each day. This is an extraordinarily large amount. Since estrogens and estrogen-like compounds can stop ovulation in extremely high doses (as in a woman's oral contraceptive), it was not surprising that the sheep were infertile.

Scientists began investigating the source of the estrogen and discovered that it was the clover grass in the pasture. These clovers, called subterranean clovers because they set their seeds under ground, had levels of isoflavones as much as 5 percent of the dry weight of the plant. Since the pasture consisted mainly of clover, the sheep were getting very large amounts of isoflavones every day.

Q. What is the connection with red clover?

A. The discovery that subterranean clovers are so rich in estrogenic isoflavones prompted scientists to start looking further. They found that other members of the clover family also have isoflavones. Red clover was found to have less than half of the amount found in the subterranean clovers but still a comparatively high amount. Because red clover is widely used throughout the world to feed dairy cows, scientists in Europe and North America then discovered that the sheep, cattle, and horses that ate red clover, especially varieties with a high isoflavone content, also showed evidence of mild estrogenic effects, though nowhere near as dramatic as that of the Australian sheep.

It was shortly after this that scientists working in England in the 1970s discovered that the same isoflavones found in the blood of sheep and cattle eating clovers were also present in the blood and urine of people eating soy. From that point, it quickly became clear that all legumes contain these isoflavones and that anyone who eats legumes in significant quantities, whether they be clover, soy, chick peas, lentils, or any one of the many different sorts of beans will have estrogenic isoflavones in his or her body.

Q. Who should take the red clover supplement?

A. Red clover is intended for women either approaching menopause or in menopause. It provides a rich source of estrogenic isoflavones for women who would rather not change their diets.

Red clover is not recommended for men or for women who are pregnant or could be pregnant.

Q. What should I look for in buying a quality red clover supplement?

A. There are several things you should look for in choosing a supplement. To start, you should pay attention to the part of the clover plant used to make the supplement. The isoflavones in red clover are found mostly in the leaves; very low levels are found in the flowers. With red clover products that are made from the flowers, you need to take a lot of tablets to get the recommended dose of about 40 mg of isoflavones.

Some quality products made from the leaves of red clover contain 40 mg of isoflavone per tablet, and most women find that one tablet per day of these products is adequate. Therefore, it is also important that you check the label for the iso-flavone level of the tablets. You want to make sure that the levels are standardized, that is, that the level of each isoflavone is guaranteed, so that you may be sure of the dosage.

You also should note whether the isoflavone dosage quoted on the label refers to isoflavones in their glycoside or free (aglycone) form. In the glyco-side form, in which they are attached to a large sugar molecule, 10 mg of isoflavone equals only 4 mg of the active, free form. If they are present in the tablet in their free form, then 10 mg means 10 mg.

Q. Will I notice results immediately?

A. It may take four or five weeks before you notice a clear response. You should continue taking the tablets even if a long time elapses in the beginning with no results. Remember, you probably have been without the benefit of appreciable levels of phytoestrogens for most of your life. You have a lot of time to make up for.

Q. Are there any side effects from red clover?

A. There are no major side effects. As with any supplement, a small number of people will report some minor side effects. A few people have reported a minor skin rash after taking red clover supplements. These people may have been allergic to one of the inactive ingredients in the particular tablet used rather than to red clover itself. The rash went away quickly when use of the supplement was discontinued. No other side effects have been reported. This very low incidence of side effects from red clover puts it in the category of a very well-tolerated product.

In the clinical trials performed by Dr. Brown described earlier, there was important safety data on red clover. No adverse side effects were reported by any of the women taking it. In particular, there was no apparent adverse effect on the endometrium (the lining the uterus). No woman reported the breakthrough bleeding that usually accompanies HRT use. Ultrasound examination failed to find any thickening of the endometrium after three months of treatment. That isoflavones do not appear to have any effect on the lining of the reproductive tract is good news for menopausal women.

Finally, red clover does not appear to have any of the anti-nutritive factors present in some other legumes, such as soy.

Q. Will I develop tender breasts after taking red clover?

A. Another important safety observation reported from the same clinical trials was that red clover supplementation was not associated with breast tenderness. In addition to stimulating the endometrium, HRT is often associated with the stimulation of breast tissue, which can increase the risk of breast cancer. Red clover appears to have no effect on the breasts. The same type of estrogen receptor that is found in the endometrium is also dominant in the breast, and isoflavones have little compatibility with this type of receptor.

Q. Will red clover make me gain weight?

A. HRT is often associated with weight gain; women typically gain seven or eight pounds within several months of starting estrogen therapy. Most of this is due to water retention in the body caused by estrogen.

Red clover has no such effect. Women in the studies mentioned above reported no weight gain over eight months of treatment. Part of this may owe to the fact that red clover is a mild diuretic. Rather than causing the body to retain water, as steroidal estrogens and progesterone do, isoflavones actually cause the body to shed water.

Another feature of red clover in this regard is that it is virtually calorie-free, unlike many other sources of isoflavones.

Q. What is the best way to store red clover supplements?

A. The isoflavones in quality red clover supplements should be fairly stable at high temperatures, but it is best to store them in a cool, dry place below 85°F. It's probably fine to carry red clover tablets in your purse for a few days, but try to avoid exposures to heat and humidity. If you live in a part of the country that's hot and humid, consider keeping your red clover supplements in the refrigerator.

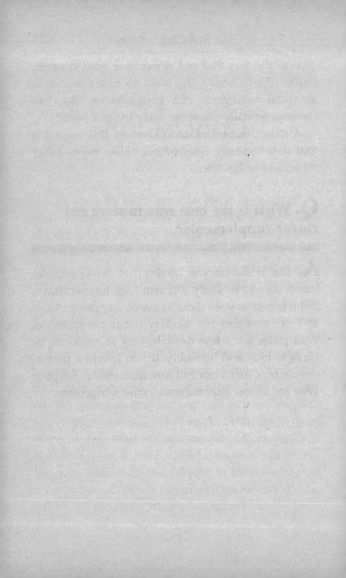

Conclusion

Contrary to what you may hear or read, menopause is neither a disease nor an "estrogen-deficiency disorder." Menopause is a natural phase of life marked by falling estrogen levels. It is inevitable that such a decline in estrogen will produce some consequences for women, but these can be made less severe in a safe way.

Many of the health problems that American women experience during menopause are the results of an inadequate diet and inadequate exercise. American women do obtain some phytoestrogens through food, but the scarcity of legumes in their diets means that they are not getting enough of the most important type of phytoestrogens, the isoflavones. If everyone had the time and the inclination to eat more legumes, then women probably would not need to supplement their diets with red clover. However, this is not the reality of today's busy world. Fortunately, red clover can fill in the gap between what women should eat and what they do eat.

The scientific research on the beneficial effects of phytoestrogens in alleviating many of the symptoms of menopause is impressive. Red clover may allow you a smooth transition into menopause without compromising the bright future you have ahead.

Glossary

Angiogenesis. The formation of new blood vessels, which facilitates the growth of solid tumors.

Biochanin. An estrogenic isoflavone found in legumes, particularly chick peas. It may have an anti-estrogenic quality with respect to human breast cells.

Cardiovascular. Refers to the circulatory system, which includes the heart, veins, and arteries.

Climacteric. An older term for menopause.

Daidzein. An estrogenic isoflavone found in legumes.

Diuretic. Any substance that encourages loss of water from the body.

Endometrium. The internal lining of the uterus (or womb).

Estradiol. The main and strongest steroidal estrogen produced by the body. It is mainly manufactured in the ovaries.

Estrogens. Female sex hormones that affect the health and activity of virtually all cells in the body. In particular, they stimulate the growth and activity of reproductive tissues. There are three main estrogens: estradiol, estrone, and estriol.

Formononetin. An estrogenic isoflavone found in legumes. It is converted in the body into daidzein.

Genistein. An estrogenic isoflavone found in legumes. It also may have strong anti-cancer activities.

HDL. High-density lipoprotein cholesterol. This is the "good" cholesterol.

Hormone. A substance found in plants and animals that works by activating a specific receptor on a cell.

Hot flash (also called hot flush). A symptom of menopause characterized by reddening of the skin around the upper body, neck, and head, along with sweating and a feeling of heat.

HRT. Hormone replacement therapy. It is comprised either of synthetic steroidal estrogen, steroidal estrogen plus progesterone, or estrogens isolated from the urine of pregnant mares.

Isoflavones. Plant substances with a phenolic-ring structure. Some isoflavones are plant hormones. Of over 1,000 isoflavones discovered, about six are estrogenic.

LDL. Low-density lipoprotein cholesterol. This is the cholesterol that has adverse effects on the cardiovascular system when present in high amounts.

Legume. A plant that has the ability to convert atmospheric nitrogen into protein. Legumes are good dietary sources of vegetable protein and isoflavones.

Menopause. The time of the last menstruation (or period).

Menstruation. The periodic (monthly) shedding of the endometrium.

Mood swings. Relatively sudden shifts (highs and lows) in personality and emotions.

Night sweats. Hot flashes at night, which are characterized by profuse sweating.

Osteoblasts. The cells in bone responsible for bone production.

Osteoclasts. The cells in bone responsible for bone destruction.

Osteoporosis. Gradual loss of density of bone, which predisposes toward fractures.

Ovulation. The maturation of a follicle in the ovary and its release as an egg.

Phytoestrogen. Naturally occurring plant substances that have estrogenic properties in animals and people.

Perimenopause. The time leading up to the last period. It is normally associated with irregularity of menstruation.

Progesterone. A steroidal hormone produced mainly by the ovaries. Its major role is maintenance of pregnancy.

Soy (also called soya). A legume used in many Eastern countries as a source of dietary protein.

Steroidal hormone. Hormones that have a chemical structure known as steroid. They are synthesized from cholesterol.

References

Adlercreutz H, "Phytoestrogens: epidemiology and a possible role in cancer protection," *Environmental Health Perspectives* 103 (supplement 7) (1995): 103–112.

Brown D, et al., "Standardized red clover extract," Natural Products Research Consultants, Seattle, Washington (1997).

Eden JA, "Phytoestrogens," Paper presented at the first Australasian Menopause Society Congress, Perth, Australia (October, 1997).

Ingram D, et al., "Case-control study of phytoestrogens and breast cancer," *Lancet* 350 (1997): 990–994.

Lock, M, "Menopause in cultural context," *Experimental Gerontology* 29 (3) (1994): 307–317.

Lock M, et al., "Cultural construction of the menopausal syndrome: 'The Japanese Case'," *Maturitas* 8 (1) (1988): 317–322.

McCullough M, "Hope or hype?" *The Philadelphia Inquirer* (May 3, 1996).

Messina M, et al., "Phytoestrogens and breast cancer," *Lancet* 350 (1997): 971–972.

Stephens FO, "Phytoestrogens and prostate cancer: possible preventive role," *Medical Journal of Australia* 167 (3) (1997): 138–140.

Suggested Readings

Lark S. *The Estrogen Decision*. Berkeley, CA: Celestialarts Publishing, 1995.

Ojeda L. *Menopause Without Medicine*. Alameda, CA: Hunter House, 1995.

Shandler N. *Estrogen the Natural Way*. New York, NY: Villard, 1997.

Stewart M. *Beat the Menopause Without HRT*. London: Headline, 1997.

Stewart M. *The Phyto Factor*. London: Vermilion, 1998.

Index

Aches, menopause and, 34
Aglycone, 72
Angiogenic inhibition, 56–57
Anti-inflammatories, 32–33, 58
Antioxidants, 32, 58, 60–62
Atherosclerosis, 31–32. *See also* Cardiovascular disease.

Biochanin, 53, 58
  benefits of, 61
  changes during absorption, 64
  sources of, 62
  See also Isoflavones; Phytoestrogens.
Bladder problems, menopause and, 34–35
Bone tissue, formation of, 26–28, 29
Bones, thinning. *See* Osteoporosis.
Breast cancer
  HRT and, 45, 47, 55, 74
  isoflavones and, 57–58
Breasts
  effects of menopause on, 22
  effects of red clover on, 74
Brown, Donald, M.D., 66

Caffeine, calcium absorption and, 29
Calcium absorption, caffeine and, 29
Candida albicans, 23
Cardiovascular disease
  effects of estrogen on, 32–33
  menopause and, 30–33
  reducing risk of, 33
Chalcones, 50
Cholesterol, 31–32, 33